Franklin Park Chiropractor Reveals:

47 Reasons to Visit Your Chiropractor

Dr. Frank J. Hahn

This publication is designed to provide
accurate and authoritative information
in regard to the subject matter covered.
It is sold with the understanding the
publisher is not engaged in rendering
legal, accounting, or other professional
services. If legal advice or other expert
assistance is required, the services of a
competent professional person should be
sought.

First Printing, 2011

ISBN-13: 978-1461050322
ISBN-10: 1461050324
Printed in the United States of America

If you have any questions or comments
for this author, please visit the author's
website:

www.MyChiroCenter.com

Table of Contents

Introduction

This book is a quick tip guide for many reasons a Chiropractor helps your body function better. We listed 47 examples how your body starts to break down from daily activities along with helpful tips to counter those stressful activities. I'm sure many of you can think of many more reasons.

From being pregnant to being born and leaning to walk, dating and dancing, cleaning your house to pulling weeds and a lot more.

Capturing everyday activities people do and explaining how stressful situations impact your daily life is the prime motivation for this book. We give you simple helpful tips and show you many ways to maintain your quality of life throughout your lifetime.

Enjoy and Be Well!

About the Author

Dr. Frank Joseph Hahn is a Doctor of Chiropractic and owner of Chiropractic LifeCenter in Franklin Park, New Jersey. Dr. Hahn earned his degree from Sherman College of Chiropractic in South Carolina in 2003. He was awarded the BJ Palmer Philosophy Award during graduation. This is a very special award for his ability to communicate and educate the public about Chiropractic Philosophy.

Dr. Hahn has enhanced the quality of many people's lives through Chiropractic care while working in private practice since he graduated. Volunteering his time away from the office he checks spines at local soup kitchens and helps educate his community at local charity events. He is committed to helping people through Chiropractic care.

Dr. Hahn served as editor for the Garden State Chiropractic newsletter, <u>Straight to You</u> for five years. Additionally he developed a 14 week internship program for future Chiropractic students in order to help grow the profession.

In May 2010 Sherman College of Chiropractic awarded Dr. Frank Hahn the Spirit of Sherman College Award, an honor presented to a Chiropractor who exemplifies the true spirit of Sherman College in his home community.

What is Chiropractic?

T he way your body works is highly complex, yet is so simple to explain.

Your brain creates and sends messages down your spinal cord, across your nerves, which exit between your spinal bones to every muscle and organ in your body. This is how your brain communicates with everything in your body and you stay alive.

Chiropractic 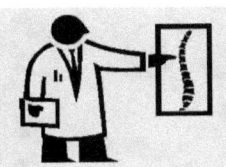 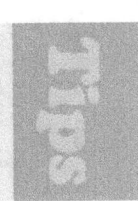 Tips

When a spinal bone moves out of position, it can place unwanted pressure on your nerves and interfere or block those vital messages that are trying to cross through your nerves. **Chiropractic is the Art, Science & Philosophy** of locating and helping to correct this spinal misalignment issue.

What Causes People to Visit Their Chiropractor?

The serious health concern called **Spinal Subluxation** (misaligned spinal bones) is the main reason one must visit a Chiropractor. Results from Spinal Subluxations include a lack of normal motion of the spinal joints; more important, misaligned bones affect the spinal nerves as they exit through the joint.

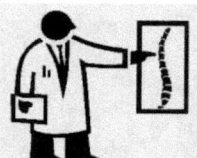

Chiropractic Tips

Chiropractic Care is vital to the removal of Spinal Subluxations. Chiropractic care helps your nervous system (brain, spinal cord, and nerves) to function optimally. Without optimal nerve flow and removal of these misaligned spinal bones it is impossible to achieve optimal health.

Pregnancy...

Pregnancy results in a **number of changes** to your body. Not only structural changes occur, you have chemical changes too. When your pelvis moves, it can place unwanted pressure on your sciatic nerve and create irritation. As your abdomen increases in size, it can increase the curve in your lower back. As your pelvis changes, your posture needs to adapt also.

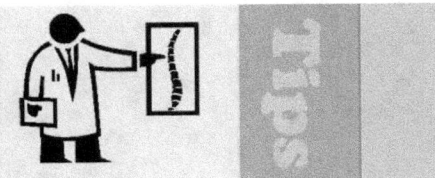

Going to a **Chiropractor throughout** your entire pregnancy can help mom's pelvis, back and neck stay in good alignment, as well as helping baby to rotate into an optimal position.

Giving Birth...

From the moment you find out you are pregnant to the **day you give birth**; you will experience many changes and learn new ways to take care of yourself and your growing baby.

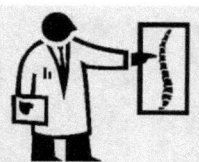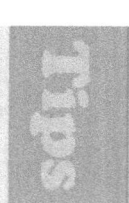

Attend a **childbirth class** and bring your spouse along! In these classes, it is often well explained how a birth actually happens, when you should call your midwife, pain relief and much more. Many of the online birthing classes are excellent too.

Being Born...

After birth, **how long should I wait** to have the little one checked for misaligned bones? Even the most natural birthing experience is somewhat traumatic to the baby and they may have misaligned spinal bones from birth.

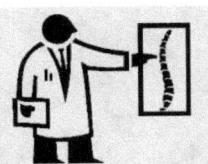 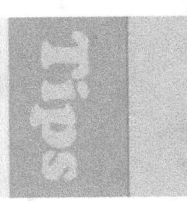

Because the little one cannot communicate like you or I yet, you won't know if they have a misaligned bone until they're checked by a Chiropractor. Have the little one checked right away. **All children function better with 100% nerve function.** All children deserve the right to express their fullest potential.

Learning to Walk...

L earning to walk is one of the most precious encounters in a child's life. As the little one comes crashing down on their backside repetitively seems somewhat harmless. Research shows the **number one reason** spinal bones misalign is repetitive stress applied to a specific joint. Sometimes, the very first misalignments we can be exposed to in life are the ups & downs learning to walk.

Chiropractic 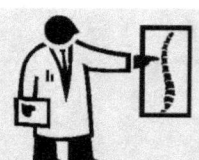 Tips

Your child's Chiropractor will apply light pressure with their fingertips during an adjustment to restore proper motion of the vertebrae and relax the muscles. If neglected, the bumps and falls during this period of rapid growth may lead to serious spinal issues later in life. This can set the stage for **scoliosis** and a **weakened immune system** response.

Kids In and Out of Car Seats...

H ave you ever noticed how much some people **strain their bodies** when placing and removing their young children to/from car seats? Bending at your hips to pick up your toddler with extended arms places extreme pressure on your joints & discs as well as strain on muscles in your back, neck and shoulders.

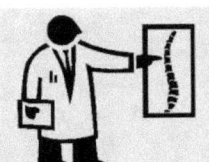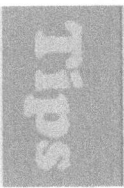

Repetition will result in misalignments of your joints. The first tip is to **decrease the strain** on the parents' body by having the child climb into their car seat on his/her own. You may have to give them a hand in the beginning, but they learn quickly. Kneel on the back seat, do not stand outside the car and try to place the child in their car seat.

Computer Time/ Video Games...

Each body position requires certain muscles to shorten and others to lengthen for **proper function**. This occurs every time we move. If we were to stay in one position for too long those muscles will eventually spasm and not function properly. When you're playing computer games for long periods of time, this will lead to spastic muscles.

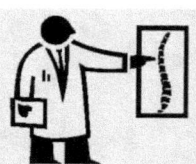

Chiropractic **Tips**

Sit on a chair and make sure your back is straight and leaning against the chair.
You can sit on the floor but try to have a support for your back.
Take a 5 minute break at least every 30-45 minutes & do some activities that involve stretching your joints. Drink some water to restore your energy.

Poor Posture...

Poor posture **stresses joints & strains muscles** which often do lead to misaligned spinal bones. When you compensate and move differently you set the stage for injury when you just "move wrong" and something "goes out". Posture compensation is a major cause of misalignments forming in your body.

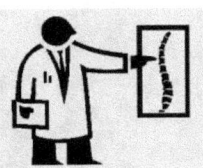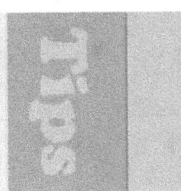

Chiropractic Tips

Once injured, the body moves to avoid pain. If it hurts to move normally but feels better to move with your body distorted, your motion will be distorted.

Over time, muscles, ligaments & nerves become trained & learn to move differently. **UNBALANCED MOTION** creates chronic postural changes within your body.

Poor Posture II...

Even **exercising** with unbalanced motion often only aggravates the problem!

Only when joints move freely through a full range of motion can weak muscles strengthen, tight muscles stretch, and ligaments adapt to balanced posture.

Chiropractic 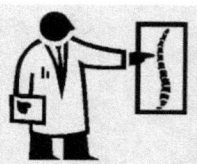 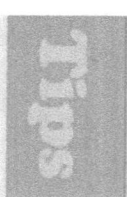 **Tips**

Balanced motion creates (and maintains) flexibility and stable posture to keep the body moving, feeling, and being well.

Restore motion to balance posture so you move naturally and **optimal performance** is achieved.

Playing Sports, Exercise & Lifting Weights...

Cardiovascular and strengthening exercises combined with Chiropractic care are important in the management of your health. Specific instructions can be given by your Chiropractor with respect to **proper exercise** for help with a patient's total health.

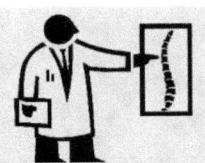 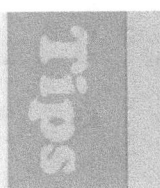

There is no one right way to move, but if you let muscles and joints stop moving, over time your overall body loses its ability to move. If you want to move well when you are old, you must keep your body moving well as you age. When you **stop moving, you stop living**, staying active is the ultimate desire of people as we age.

Talking on the Cell Phone...

Everywhere you go you are likely to see **someone talking on a cell phone**.

Think about how many surfaces you touch throughout the day ~ door handles, hand rails, elevator buttons and ATM screens. Now consider how many times you touch your cell phone before washing your hands. Gross, right?

Chiropractic 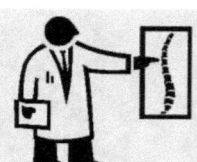 Tips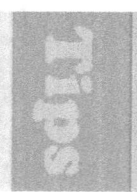

The good news is we can break this gross cycle by getting in the habit of **spring cleaning our cell phones** all year-round in order to stave off germs and bacteria.

Don't use any harsh chemicals, or even more damaging ~ NO water. Use a cleaner like iKlear along with a microfiber cloth.

Dating...

S ure dating in this day and age is stressful. If you **love dating or hate it**, even bad dates are kind of fun. Hey, at least you get a good story out of it! But for a lot of people, new relationships are super nerve-racking and filled with anxiety. If these emotions sound familiar, here is some advice that will help you cope and remain sane.

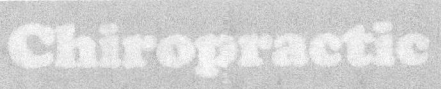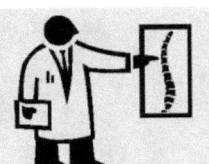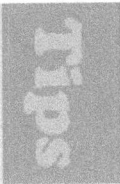

Anxiety is like the ocean tide. Once it starts coming, the waves keep rolling in, and once it starts to recede, it keeps going out.
If you've already met your date, then the hard part is already over. Very few things in life are so important that you can't laugh about them later.
Remember to Laugh A LOT!

Dancing...

Professional **dancers** are among the hardest working of all athletes. This work puts a lot of stress on your body, muscles become strained and bones can become misaligned. People who want to excel and perform at an elite level or simply want a night out on the town can each benefit from having your bones checked for misalignments.

Chiropractic 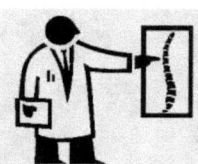 **Tips**

Dancing is a fun substitute for boring exercise programs while allowing you to be as energetic as you like. Social levels of dancing burn from 100-400 calories/hr, while competitive **dancers burn up to 600+ calories/hr.** Two to three hours of continuous social dancing can give you an excellent low-impact aerobic workout.

Studying For Exams...

I t's that season again! Sore throats, runny noses, and headaches; No it's not Winter or Spring, its **Final Exam Season** again. Did you ever notice students getting run down right after the BIG exam? There are a variety of ways to fight getting run down symptoms and stay healthy. Here are a few ways to stay energized during the stressful exam season.

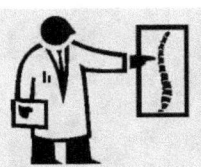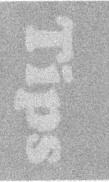

Eat Smarter – Breakfast is a must & donuts just don't cut it. You need protein, calcium, fiber and a piece of fruit or a vegetable.
Lack of Sleep impairs memory and alertness; Compensate by taking a nap in the afternoon.
Stay Well Hydrated. Choose your beverages well avoid caffeine, replace with water or fruit juice.

Vacation & Long Car Rides...

Family's vacationing now may ultimately decide to **travel by car rather than air** and that doesn't have to throw a wrench in your summer travels. In fact, if you keep the following tips in mind, you may very well make your trip a comfortable one.

Chiropractic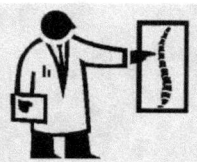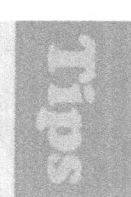

Bring a pillow or back support and place it between your lower back and seat for some extra support. Don't sit on your wallet, cell phone or anything else that may throw your spine out of whack.

Make it a point to spend a couple of minutes doing **back exercises at a rest stop** before getting back on the road.

Riding a Horse...

An estimated **30 million Americans ride horses** each year. However, more than 2,300 riders under the age of 25 years are hospitalized annually because of horseback-riding injuries. The most frequent types of injuries are bruises, strains, and sprains, which affect the soft tissues (skin, ligaments, tendons, and muscles). Other types of injuries include fractures (broken bones), dislocations, and Subluxations.

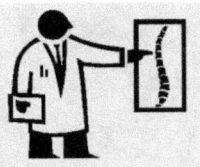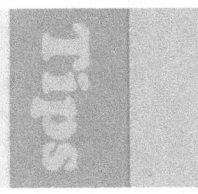

Hard shell helmets should be worn at all times when mounted. Riders should wear properly fitted boots and nonskid gloves. **Proper gear** can be used to prevent soft tissue injuries; however, it does not protect the spine from injury. Always have your spine checked for misaligned spinal bones after every ride.

Carrying Luggage...

L uggage might be the last thing you think about when it comes to **safety measures** for your next vacation but don't risk hurting yourself before you even arrive at your destination. Here is some full-proof ways of making sure your luggage doesn't end up holding you back from your travel destination.

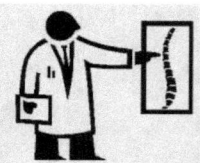 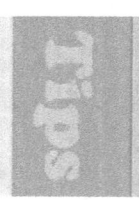

Do not load **too much stuff** in one luggage; preferably break them down in several luggage or bags. Remember, you usually bring back more items than you start with.
Select a **wheeled luggage** or backpack.
Be very careful when **lifting luggage** to place it higher than your head.

A Strange Bed...

Beds can really help one have a good night's sleep and wake up feeling **rested and refreshed**. Sleeping on an unusual bed can cause sleeplessness, back pain, and overall aches and pains. For people with a back problem, a bed that isn't a good fit can make the body function worse.

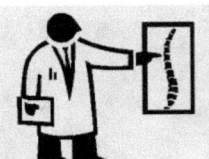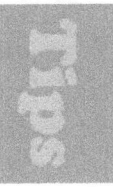

If comfort is not the only thing making sleep difficult and if anyone experiences significant or persistent back pain, there may be an **underlying back condition** that has nothing to do with the mattress. It is always advisable for people to consult with a health care provider for a thorough exam and treatment program.

Over Eating...

Sights, Sounds, and Smells. Overeating can be triggered by the alluring smell of bacon cooking, the sound of popcorn popping, advertisements for junk food, and so on. You are influenced by your surroundings, and studies show these kinds of cues result in eating more food.

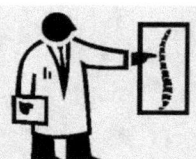

Chiropractic Tips

According to researchers, in addition to keeping the organs of the body functioning properly, helping the musculoskeletal system to stay strong and mobile, and burning calories for weight loss, **Chiropractic with exercise** has also been found to restore the sensitivity of neurons involved in control of *satiety* ("feeling full").

Carrying a Backpack...

Backpacks come in all sizes, colors, fabrics, and shapes and help children of all ages express their own personal sense of style. And when used properly, they're incredibly handy. When worn correctly, the weight in a backpack is **evenly distributed** across the body, and shoulder and neck injuries are less common.

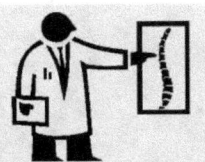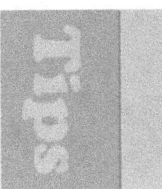

Some children have backaches because they're lugging around their entire locker's worth of books & school supplies all day long. Research recommends that children carry no more than **10% to 15%** of their body weight in their packs.

Doing Laundry...

When most people think of areas of safety concerns in the home, the **laundry room** is not the first place to come to mind. However, laundry rooms are where toxic soaps, chemicals and bleach are often stored. Dryer lint is highly combustible and many home fires begin in laundry rooms. Make your home laundry room a safer place by practicing simple safety procedures.

 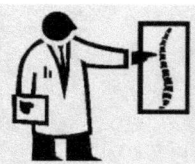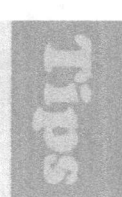

Cleaning solutions and chemical mixtures should be stored in their original containers. Clean the lint filter on the dryer to prevent fires. Pay attention and watch your step when carrying laundry, especially if you use stairs. It is safer to **carry two smaller loads** so you can see and avoid tripping.

Waiting Tables...

T he duties of a waitress may seem simple, but until you have **walked a 12 hour shift in their shoes**, don't be so sure the job is easy. Waitresses handle the customer visits in total. They may have to provide the customer with service when something is not right with their meal. Waitresses need to follow safety standards and food safety requirements. They must work as a team helping to keep the dining facilities clean.

 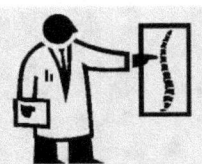 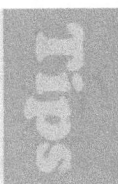

The environment can be stressful.

Find a comfortable pair of non slip shoes. Purchase a pair of shoe inserts for more protection of your feet and back. Practice balancing your tray on both sides of your shoulders to avoid those chronic joint breakdowns from repeat stress to one joint.

Carrying Groceries...

When you don't have a car and you usually **walk to the grocery store**, the dilemma of how to carry your groceries home can be a real problem. But there is no reason to worry. There are a few steps that you can take to make it home with all of your groceries easily.

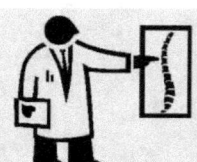 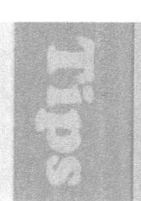

Chiropractic Tips

Choose the **correct grocery bag** for your needs. Plastic or paper bags with handles or a fabric tote bag may also work well because it will be easy to carry and it's environmentally friendly.
Consider using a grocery bag grip. Buy a collapsible cart if you have a lot of groceries to carry home.

Cleaning Your House..

Regular home cleaning such as dusting, sanitizing and picking objects off the floor makes a home safer. But the **home cleaning process** itself should be safe too; mixing chemicals and using unstable perches to change light bulbs does not promote safe cleaning. Follow the proper lifting technique for heavy objects: bend and lift with the legs and avoid twisting at the waist.

 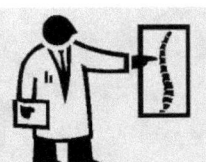 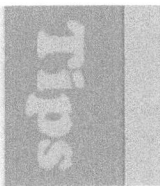

Use a ladder to reach high spots & wear slip-resistant shoes. **Caution others** the floor is wet after mopping to avoid people getting injured from slipping and falling.

Painting Your Ceiling..

C eilings are the most difficult areas to paint, but well worth the effort.

Many hazards include: Ladders, platforms & scaffolds, slips, trips & falls. Exposure to paint chemicals, working in awkward positions & performing repetitive physical tasks including heavy lifting & standing long periods of time place major stresses on your spine.

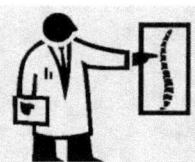

Chiropractic Tips

Work involving movement repeated over and over is very tiring because the **worker cannot fully recover** in the short periods of time between movements. Eventually, it takes more effort to perform the same repetitive movements. When the work activity continues in spite of the fatigue, injuries occur.

Walking Your Dog...

Dogs have been **"man's best friend"** for thousands of years. Since dogs watch over their owners, it's our responsibility as dog-loving humans to return the favor and keep them safe at all times. If there's anything that all dogs love to do, it's walk. They always get a thrill from each of the new smells, sounds, and sights, as well as the other animals, dogs, and people they encounter along the way.

 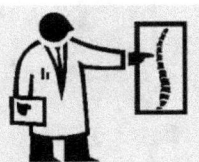 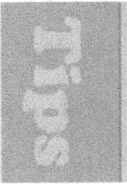

Most expert dog walkers will agree the best leash is a six foot leather lead.

Try not allowing your dog to **yank on your arm or shoulder** very hard as this could misalign joints. Keep weather in mind whenever you're walking. If it's too hot, the dog can overheat, and if it's too cold, frostbite is a serious risk.

Giving the Dog a Bath

Most dogs seem to **love outdoor water**, especially larger breeds. Sometimes getting a bath at home is another story. You'll want to bathe your dog every four weeks or so, and for some dogs who like to play in the mud and spend lots of time in the great outdoors, perhaps even more often.

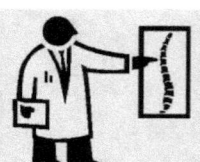 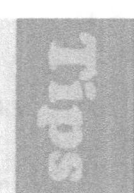

Chiropractic Tips

With many dogs, the bath is made easier with a hand-held showerhead, otherwise, use a large pitcher. **You will get wet and soapy** along with your dog, so wear old clothes. If it is a warm summer day, an outdoor bath is just fine. Consider warming up a pail of water if it is not really hot out so the dog does not get chilly.

Working on the Car...

Auto mechanic is a potentially dangerous job. **Car repairs can also be fun and very rewarding**. To keep the fun and rewards you need to prevent accidents by working safely. Many do-it-yourself mechanics are injured every year, while performing repairs at home.

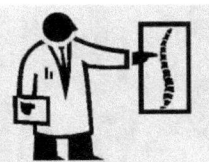 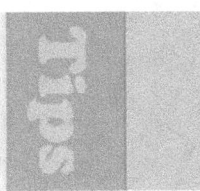

Keep the floor clean ~ clutter and mess are the first enemies of safety.

Make Safety a Priority ~ Safety is synonymous with planning, meaning that if you plan your work area and task ahead, your safety will be insured.

Driving in Heavy Traffic...

D riving for **long periods of time** or during a stressful daily commute can be especially tough on your body. Tilting to the side or leaning your head forward to much, rounded shoulders, slouching upper & lower back all add high amounts of stress on your spine.

Chiropractic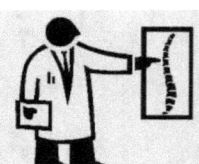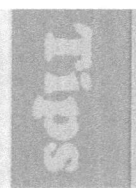

Sit firmly against the seat. Car seats do not provide much back support, try placing a pillow or a back support cushion.
Be sure you're not sitting on anything that would throw your spine out of alignment (such as a wallet in your back pocket).
Take Breaks ~ Pull over every two hours and stretch.

Car Accidents...

If you had a car accident and you have any doubts about your health, you need to **see a Chiropractor immediately**. Don't wait to see if symptoms arise or trust that because "you're still fine now" that you'll stay this way. It's worth your time and money to get a piece of mind that you are actually fine after your accident.

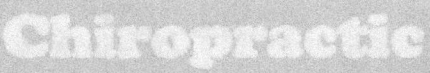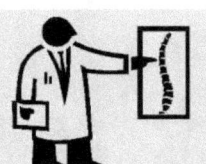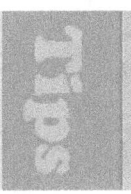

No matter how minor we believe the impact from a car accident, the minor force is enough pressure on your spine to **misalign a spinal bone**. Once the bone is on the nerve, it can block the signals from the brain to the body parts. This causes your body not to function properly whether you can measure it right now or later in life.

Mowing the Lawn...

Each year hundreds of Americans are badly injured while mowing their lawns. Most of these accidents occur because of **improper use of lawn mowers**, heat stroke and lifting problems.

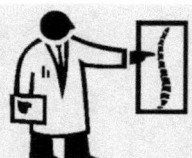

Making adjustments to your mower should always be done while the blade is off. Never wear sandals while mowing lawns. Lawn mowing is a physically demanding activity and your body will not function properly without plenty of water. **Safety should always be your first priority** while mowing lawns.

Pulling Weeds...

G ardening can provide a great workout, but with all the bending, twisting, reaching and pulling, your body may not be ready for exercise of the garden variety. **Gardening can be enjoyable** and it's important to stretch your muscles too before reaching for your gardening tools.

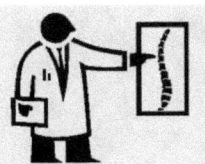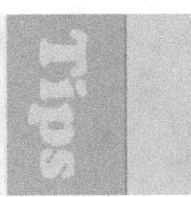

While sitting, keeping the knees straight, lean forward until you feel a stretch in the back of the leg. **Stand** and pull one heel towards your buttocks with hand and hold the position for 15 seconds. **Remain standing**, weave your fingers together above your head palms up. Lean to one side for 10 seconds, then the other.

Bending Over...

Have you ever heard of this issue? I just bent over one ill-fated time and I cannot stand straight. In reality, this problem most likely stems from years of an **unstable spine**. You have heard it before. "Bend your knees when you pick that up or you'll hurt your back." Well, that's true, to a degree. The fact is simply bending your knees is not enough to prevent low back injury.

Chiropractic 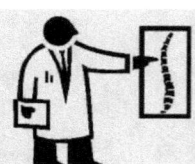 **Tips**

The first step in lifting an object is to stand close to it and make sure it is right in line with your belly button. The second step is tilting your pelvis forward to lock the low back. If the object is too large, drop to a knee before lifting. My last piece of advice in regards to lifting is very easy to remember. **If it's too heavy, get help with it!**

Sneezing...

Did you know that a sneeze or cough can have a **speed of 40 to 167 mph?** If you think about it, your body has to withstand plenty of forces by contracting and bracing the spine and the surrounding muscles. The force of a cough or sneeze can misalign spinal bones enough to create pressure on your nerves.

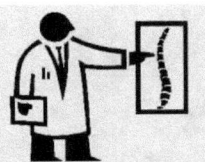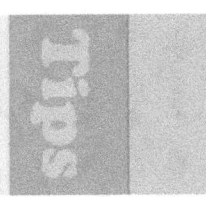

Remember, Chiropractors are not treating you for specific symptoms when we adjust your spine, we need to **free up those vital messages** from your brain that must get through all those nerve pathways to allow your body to function properly.

Sitting in a Tree While Hunting...

Homemade tree stands is rated up at the **top of the list** when it comes to hunters falling. Often these types of stands can only handle a few years out in the elements before the boards and steps start coming loose.

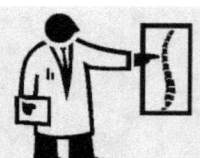 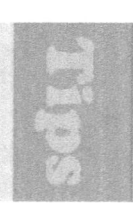

Instead of using regular lumber to build your tree stand, use **Pressure Treated Lumber** to withstand longer exposure in the elements.
Always replace old and worn out parts of your tree stand with new.

Moving Furniture...

Moving is not only emotionally difficult, but your body can also **undergo a lot of stress** with minor and more severe injuries a possibility. Even if you're hiring a moving company, you need to make sure that your home is safety-proofed.

Chiropractic 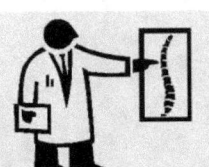 Tips

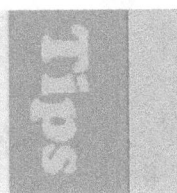

When packing, make sure all boxes weigh less than 50 pounds.
Rent proper equipment to save back strain and to help move larger, heavier pieces.
Organize the space so the high-traffic areas are clear of any obstacles.

Couch Potato Syndrome...

T here you are, sitting on the couch again, watching TV instead of exercising. You know you should get up and get to the gym, or even just take a brisk walk around the block, but something's stopping you. You're deep in the clutches of the evil **Couch Potato Syndrome.**

Chiropractic 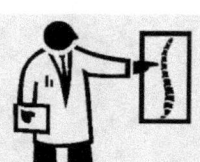 **Tips**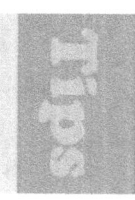

Physical inactivity is a major contributor to heart disease, osteoporosis, adult-onset diabetes and cancer. **Moderate Exercise** can be easy and fun to integrate into everyday life, and can include activities such as biking, walking, swimming... even gardening. Get off that couch and do something about your health.

Fixing the Toilet...

I f your toilet is clogged and will not flush, what do you do?
Common sense says grab your plunger and unclog it. What if that doesn't work? Lift the lid to the tank and see if the components are connected properly. Next, try pouring some unclogging liquid and you usually find that stuff doesn't work either.

You need to call on a professional PLUMBER.

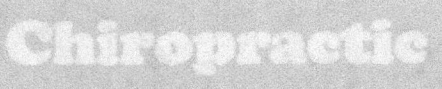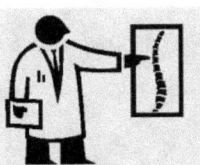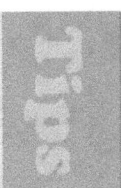

When your bones misalign and your brains messages are not getting through properly to your body, what are the odds you're going to be able to correct these misalignments all on your own?
You can try other methods.

You need to call on a professional CHIROPRACTOR.

Fixing the Shower Head...

This might be one of the most routine things we do: take a shower. Most people notice when water pressure is right or water is beating on them too soft or too hard. We get used to our shower and want it a certain way. Well, there might not be anything wrong with the water pressure at all **you may need to adjust your shower head**.

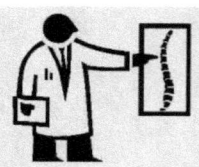

Chiropractic Tips

This is similar to your own body; we know when we are doing great and when we just aren't functioning well. There may be nothing wrong with your internal organs or systems **you may just need to be adjusted** so the communication within your body flows properly.

Physical Stress...

Stress is the **Number One reason** your bones misalign. The stress you put on yourself each day can make your muscles strain and then spasm. A muscle that spasms can misalign a spinal bone and the whole process of nerve interference begins.

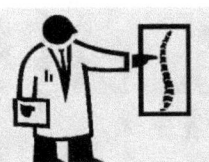 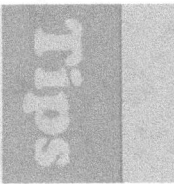

Chiropractic   Tips

Physical Stress is easy to understand, these are your slips, falls, accidents & traumas that will lead to misaligning spinal bones.

Learn ways to decrease your stress levels and your spinal bones may misalign less often.

Pain...

Pain is a great motivator to get you to do something about your health. Pain signals are really **just messages from your brain** to a damaged tissue in your body. The message is, "begin the healing process" (Inflammatory Response). Inflammation is simply blood flow, oxygen & nutrients in abundance to the damaged tissue.

Chiropractic 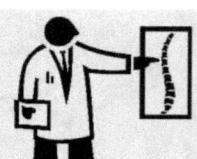 **Tips**

Pain Messages are a vital part of healing so you do need these signals to heal. No one likes to be in pain, but just know your body cannot heal up without these messages getting through the nerves to the specific body part.

Chemical Stress...

C hemical stress is any imbalance in the **chemical processes of the body**. Examples of chemical stresses on our bodies are dehydration, digestive imbalances, deficiencies in vitamins and minerals, acute and chronic infections, heavy metal toxicity, and blood sugar imbalances.

Chiropractic 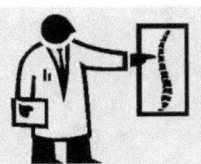 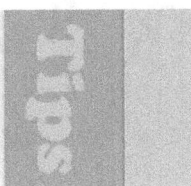 **Tips**

If we have too much stress in our life we become overwhelmed. Very few patients recognize how much chemical stress is contributing to their health concern.

The best defense against Chemical Stress is a **properly balanced diet along with proper exercise**.

Drugs...

Many drugs work in this way; they try to **eliminate the symptom** you are experiencing. There is definitely a time and a place for drugs. We're programmed almost from birth to think, "If we have a symptom, get rid of it at all costs."

Most "Symptoms" are merely a way for your immune system to defend against a foreign bacteria/virus that invaded your body.

Chiropractic 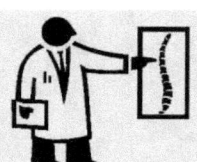 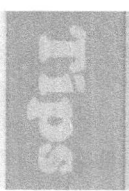 Tips

When you take any drug to decrease or eliminate your symptom it makes your body work harder to eliminate the invader. Sometimes the invader will manifest and create more problems. We should try to **strengthen our body and boost our immune system**, not just try to eliminate our symptom.

Mental Stress...

Mental stress is what most people think about when you say the word stress. However, it is not as simple as what people think. Your **Nervous System** allows you to prepare for danger by raising your blood pressure, heart rate and respiration. It also decreases blood flow to the digestive organs and increases blood flow to the muscles to prepare for Fight or Flight responses.

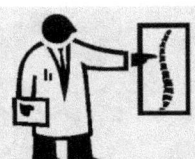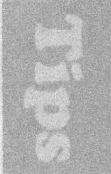

Chiropractic adjustments allow your **Body and Brain to communicate better** thus allowing your body to handle emotional states and changes in life more effectively and efficiently.

Weakened Immune System...

Our nervous system is housed within our spine, and governs all the functions of our body, including those controlled by our immune system, such as the spleen, thymus gland, lymph nodes and all other organs as well.

So how can your Chiropractor help boost your immune system?

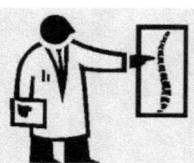

Chiropractic Tips

While you are living under continuous stress, staying free of subluxations, allows your **immune system to function at its highest** level. Along with proper Rest, Nutrition & Exercise, your Chiropractor will help keep your spine interference free.

Grandchildren...

Grandchildren are very precious. If you're lucky, you'll be able to take your grandchildren places from an early age. There's a **whole world of attractions** your own children loved that you want to introduce the grandkids. The contributions grandparents can make to their families are extraordinary. Will you be able to walk them around the Zoo? Walk with them on sand at the beach? Through the Museum?

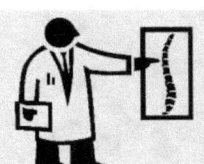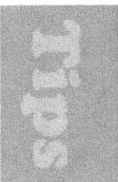

The major point, **Chiropractic care helps improve the quality of your life** by improving the function of your body. Have your spine checked as soon as you can for misaligned joints that may cause your body to break down prematurely.

Just Living...

There is a serious health issue called Spinal Subluxation. A **Spinal Subluxation** is a vertebra (spinal bone) that has stopped moving normally. As a result of the lack of normal motion, the spinal joints and discs develop degenerative changes. More importantly, the Spinal Subluxation affects the spinal nerves that exit between the vertebrae causing interference between your brain & body parts.

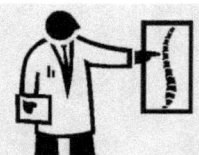

Chiropractic Tips

Doctors of Chiropractic check family's everyday in our offices, **Newborns through Seniors** and everyone in between. Make it a point to call your local Chiropractor today and make a family wellness trip to see if anyone in your family has this issue called Spinal Subluxation. Chiro~Care will make a difference.